RENAL DIET COOKBOOK

Low Sodium, Low Potassium and Low Phosphorus Healthy Recipes to Managing Kidney Diseases and Avoid Dialysis

SUSAN SHELTON

TABLE OF CONTENT

INTRODUCTION TO THE RENAL DIET!

A renal diet is an eating plan conceived to help people who suffer from renal diseases. It can expand the effectiveness of treatment by lowering the level of waste products in their blood.

This diet is designed to avoid stressing kidneys, and it provides useful nutrients and energy to the body.

The diet is based on some basic rules.

The main rule is that it must be a healthy and balanced diet, rich in fibers, natural grains, carbohydrates, omega 3 fats, vitamins and fluids. Protein should be present but not excessively, they are essential to rebuild tissues but cannot be exceeding in this diet as excessive quantities of proteins should be broken down by the body into carbohydrates and nitrates. Moreover, as nitrates are not used by the body, they should be excreted through the kidneys.

Salts are kept to a minimum and electrolyte levels of blood are checked on a regular basis and are then balanced accordingly. Please inform your doctor before starting the diet.

Carbohydrates are important for energy and need to be taken in the right quantities. However, you should avoid refined ones. You should try to use as many whole grains and unrefined forms of carbohydrates as possible.

Table salt should be used only for cooking and remember that excessive salt causes retention and stress to the kidneys. Salty foods should be avoided as well: no sausages, no snacks, no tinned food.

There is also the level of phosphorus which needs to be monitored carefully, avoiding colored drinks like colas and food with a high level of potassium such as bananas, citrus fruits, apricots, dark leafy green vegetables should be avoided too, especially if blood levels rise.

Take into consideration also Omega 3 fats which are important in your diet but avoid trans-fats and hydrolyzed fats.

The proper renal diet can really help kidneys functioning longer, and it has only more restrictions on proteins and table salt, while restrictions to phosphorous and potassium can be needed if the levels of blood rise and the signs of accumulation become too evident.

Hereafter we are going to have a look at the benefits and dangers in many foods and nutrients.

FOOD AND NUTRIENTS IN THE RENAL DIET

Protein: the best you can do is to talk to your doctor when it comes to dealing with proteins in your diet, as their presence could vary according to physical activity levels and, in any case, you should limit your protein intake if your kidneys are damaged. We still need some protein so we need to chose which are the best: cut dairy and red meat, as they are often too high in fats and sodium.

Chicken is better than red meat, but organic chicken is preferable in general. Fish is a fundamental source of proteins, and it is strong in anti-inflammatory action, which is beneficial to your kidneys.

Also soy and tofu are recommended: when taken on a regular basis, they even show a slow progression of kidney damage.

There are also three minerals which need to be avoided in your diet as kidneys need to filter the blood of these minerals to achieve the correct levels, but when kidneys are damaged this does not happen correctly, so the levels can higher and become too dangerous: potassium, phosphorus, and sodium. We will try to understand how each of these minerals can be dangerous and how to avoid them.

More in general, all diets should avoid excessive levels of sodium, as it increases blood pressure, which is a direct cause of kidneys diseases as it forces the kidneys to filter more, increasing their stress. And more kidney pressure causes high blood pressure, so this is like a dangerous circle.

Do not salt your food too much, avoid fast foods and takeaways, as they use salt a lot to increase flavor, but this is dangerous for your health. There are also foods containing hidden quantities of sodium such as processed meats, frozen and canned food, sports drinks, and snacks.

Potassium then is very important for us as it is required for nerve, cardiac functions, and fluid balance, but when its level is not the right one in our body, this may be a danger for kidneys functions. Potassium level builds up in the blood level and may end up with cardiovascular problems. We consequently need to reduce potassium in the renal diet, and we can verify this by blood sampling. We will need then to reduce the use of tomatoes, potatoes, bananas, nuts, seeds, chocolate, pumpkin, and avoid some vegetables or remove it from plants.

Phosphorus is another vital mineral for bones and teeth as it is key to the regulation of calcium, but for people suffering from kidneys damages the excessive presence of it in the blood can lead to osteoporosis and high blood pressure.

Basically, the renal diet is like an alkaline diet, as there is a need to balance pH in the blood, which is not well balanced when there is kidney disease. There is a need to avoid acidic foods from the diet. It is also true that acidity contributes to many health issues such as kidney stones, urinary problems, high blood pressure, and reduced immunity levels.

Sometimes, however, with the alkaline diet, it is not so easy to determine which foods are really acidic: let's take the lemon, for example. It tastes acidic, but it produces a real alkaline effect once it is digested.

It is right to think that most foods that are considered unhealthy are also acidic (meat, sugary treats, alcohol, wheat, most dairy products), but some acidic foods are right in the renal diet (for example olive oil, fish, soymilk, and nuts).

Following the alkaline diet, you need to consume 80% of alkaline products and 20% of acidic foods. You can, of course, test your urinary health and pH every day and then change this balance with a 60% alkaline and 40% acid.

Most alkaline foods are considered suitable for the renal diet, and they are fruits, vegetables, brown rice, green juices, tofu, sprouts, herbal teas.

The essential renal diet is crucial to your kidneys' health and to protect them from any possible future damage, and you can also add herbs and nutrients which can improve kidneys' health.

A DIET FOR PATIENTS WITH RENAL PROBLEMS

This diet is highly recommended for patients with renal problems, and what we know is that only 25% of nephrons are needed to maintain healthy renal functions. That is, it takes a long time before a kidney disease may appear, but it is also true that when we have symptoms, it means that true kidney damage is already happening.

Nitrogenous waste products, impaired excretion of electrolytes, vitamin deficiencies, and continued catabolism are the main reasons for continuous diet adjustments. Wasting syndrome is the main problem. Clients with renal issues consistently lose weight; they low down muscle mass and lose adipose tissues.

The goal in this type of nutrition is to maintain a balance of electrolytes, minerals, fluids. Dialysis on its own is not able to remove and filter the wastes in the body. The body needs to be helped in managing the accumulated waste.

The regulation of sodium, for example, is very important. When kidneys waste salt, sodium must be risen to replace it. When kidneys retain sodium, so the fluid status must be monitored to get the right info on sodium needs.

Patients and family members' quality of life are always badly affected by renal problems and therapies. All the therapies such as dialysis or also hemodialysis can affect the psychological aspects of life.

What you will find hereafter is not simply a diet but a careful analysis to approach the symptoms of renal disease and to maintain good energy levels for your daily activities. There is also information about the exact amount of proteins, electrolytes, minerals, and fluids allowed for the patients.

GUIDELINES FOR A GOOD RENAL DIET

Hereafter you will find indications on the quantity of salt to be introduced in your blood to control these levels through the food you eat. Every patient is different, and this depends on the severity of the malfunctioning, on the fact that you might be overweight or on the electrolytes in your blood: all these factors must be taken into consideration to understand if you need dialysis or not. When there is renal failure, the levels of salt in our blood can become really critical, without balance the renal diet should help you restore this balance and put your kidneys less under stress.

Renal diet guidelines are based on blood test results and on a healthy balanced diet. It tries to limit the quantity of salt intake. Fluids also are restricted if your kidneys are unable to excrete sufficient water. Proteins as well are at the minimum in order for the urea wastes to be kept low.

The salts that need to be less used and be restricted are:

Sodium, which causes high blood tension and fluid retention. There is the need for "no added salt" recipes, so you should avoid processed food, sausages, sauce, ketchup, and many canned foods.

Phosphorus cannot be removed by dialysis so it can be a big problem. Its levels must be constantly kept under control by diet and medication. So you should avoid dairy products, beans, peas, beer and cola drinks.

Potassium needs to be restricted if its level in the blood is high. So you should avoid apricots, orange juice, bananas, avocados, beets, spinach, and others.

Proteins should only be taken in small quantities. You should avoid meat, fish, eggs, and dairy products.

Fluids can be restricted if there is water retention. You should thus avoid too high quantities of beverages, soups, water, and juices.

Carbohydrates are energy food and should not be eliminated unless you are diabetic or overweight. You should also take vitamins and antioxidant supplements to help the immune system.

The renal diet is meant to decrease the workload on damaged kidneys and to maintain their health and function. It is imperative in this case to consult your doctor.

RENAL DISEASE AND THE DIET

Consult your doctor as often as you can: the kidneys are your body toxin's filter, and you should always try to clean your blood from toxins and preservatives in food.

Try not to eat irresponsibly (foods, drinks and even the air you breath) as many elements can be turned into something bad like formaldehyde due to a chemical reaction and morphing phase, which can lead to renal failure, cancer or various other problems.

Renal failure happens when your kidneys are not able to get rid of toxins and wastes in your blood, and this is called chronic kidney disease" or "chronic renal failure."

This is a progressive problem, and it can be found out, treated, the diet changed, and it might also be possible to resolve what is the cause of the problem. It usually takes a long time to get to renal failure and you certainly to want to reach it because this would require dialysis treatments to save your life, to clean the blood and remove the toxins in the blood using a machine because your body can no longer do this job. Without treatments, you could die a very painful death. It can be the result of long periods of high blood pressure, irresponsible diet, diabetes.

The renal diet uses a low quantity of proteins and phosphorus, sodium, and this will control the toxins in your blood, helping your kidneys functions. If you adjust your diet very fast and early, you could prevent total renal failure.

THE RENAL DIET FOR DIABETIC PATIENTS

For diabetics who suffer from renal disease, there is a specific diet known as diabetic renal diet. Very often, this diet is also conceived for diabetics who want to avoid incurring in renal diseases.

Diabetics and patients with renal disease often have problems in eating the right food.

The aim of this diet is to have glucose levels within the right range. This is possible by not missing any meals, by having a regular diet, by eating low glycemic carbohydrates, in order to help the body always have the same level of glucose and low glycemic foods are grains bread, sweet potatoes, and brown rice. However, if the diet is for renal problems, you should also avoid sweet potatoes and grain bread, as they are rich in potassium.

People with renal problems, as we have already seen, should avoid food rich in potassium phosphorus and sodium. Since sodium is often present, patients should look carefully at labels, and dietitians should advise patients to avoid sodas with dark colors, coffee, and drinks with too much sodium for diabetics with renal problems.

Unsweetened teas, water, and clear diet sodas are allowed. As for vegetables, broccoli, cauliflowers, beets, eggplant, and cabbage are recommended for their vitamin-rich features, together with their low potassium and carbohydrates content. You should then avoid meat such as sausage, bacon, and organ meats.

Also, avoid canned vegetables as they are rich in sodium: nutritionists will also guide you on portion sizes to help your blood glucose control.

Many people suffering from renal problems also have diabetes. The main goal for diabetic diets is to maintain the right level of glucose in your blood. This can be done by:

- Eating carbohydrates with a low glycemic index (GI) such as grains, unrefined foods, most fruits and vegetables, legumes, sweet potatoes (only in some quantities), nuts.
- White bread, sugar, confectionaries, drinks with added sugar should be avoided
- Eating small frequent meals is a good habit. Don't go long periods without eating and don't do huge meals or even worse, do not skip meals.

The renal diet then tries not to stress kidneys, and this can be done by:

- Limiting daily intake of proteins: an excess of proteins need to be broken into carbohydrates and nitrites which, in the form of urea, can be destroyed by urine as it causes stress on already damaged kidneys.

- Limiting table salt and do not use a salt replacement as they contain potassium.

- Reduce also potassium and phosphates, including apricots, avocado, bananas, kiwi, watermelon, peaches, prunes as phosphorus avoid legumes, dairy products, dried legumes, shellfish, organ meats.

The renal diet for diabetics food pyramid:

This is a pyramid (divided into 5 groups) which indicates appropriate eating, where the larger group is made up of grains, rice, beans, starchy vegetables. Then we have a smaller group including fruits and vegetables

A smaller quantity is dedicated to food with less fat and salt. If you drink alcohol, take it in moderate quantities. Choose food high in fibers and vitamins and minerals, such as whole grain and be physically active at least 30 minutes a day.

THE RENAL DIET FOR DIABETICS
FOOD PYRAMID

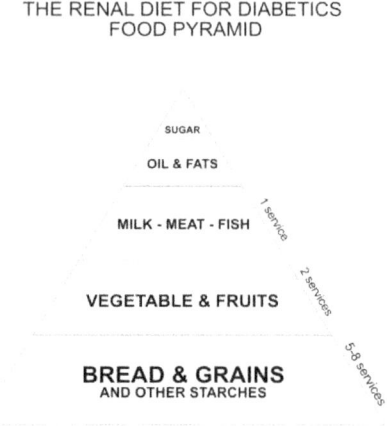

SUGAR

OIL & FATS

MILK - MEAT - FISH 1 service

VEGETABLE & FRUITS 2 services

BREAD & GRAINS
AND OTHER STARCHES 5-8 services

Eat frequently with small and repeated meals, when you wake up in the morning eat your first meal and then every 2-3 hours, taking your last meal at bedtime.

PLEASE NOTE:

If you plan your full week it will be easier for you to follow the diet, always fill up the plate with half of it with vegetables and salads, then the other half with proteins or carbohydrates.

No salt, and instead of it use fresh herbs, spices, onions, garlic, lemon juice.

For smaller meals eat whole grain cereals, crackers or bread, fruit, a glass of skim milk, nuts, yogurt, plenty of salads, or a small quantity of cottage cheese.

This diet can be powerful in both controlling renal failure and diabetes. Stick to your diet, and you will feel better and healthier.

HOW TO MANAGE DIABETES AND RENAL DISEASES EFFECTIVELY

Diabetic renal diet is a subject of interest as diabetes mellitus is one of the most common extrarenal diseases affecting the kidneys.

Diabetes mellitus leads to diabetic nephropathy in 30% of cases and to its end stage.

Researchers estimate that 25-30% of diabetes mellitus patients end up with end-stage renal diseases 10 to 20 years beginning insulin therapy.

Renal disease can also happen to non-insulin dependent diabetic patients. The incidence of protein in urine presence is about 25% after 20 years of diabetes.

The diabetic renal diet is conceived to help metabolic control in these types of patients. By controlling diabetes mellitus, we can also control the worsening situation of kidneys and prevent end-stage renal disease.

The kidney metabolizes 30-40% of insulin, and as the renal functions decline, the degradation of insulin also decreases, leading to a lower insulin need. Renal failure can be identified when the patient is evaluated for recurrent insulin reactions.

Renal disease can be controlled by
- checking hypertension carefully
- adjusting insulin therapy
- restricting protein in your diet.

However, renal failure appears within 5 to 10 years after the first appear of proteinuria (protein in urine).

The following are some recommendations for patients with diabetes mellitus.

- total calories: to maintain reasonable weight in adults, meet increased needs in children, adolescents, pregnant and lactating women and people recovering from catabolic illness

- caloric distribution: 50 to 70 % of carbohydrates, 20 to 30% of proteins, 20 to 30% of fats
- cholesterol limited under 300mg/day or less
- sodium below 300mg/day less for people with hypertension and renal complications
- alcohol: a very moderate amount

- vitamin and mineral supplements: to be given to individuals with low caloric diets (1200 kcal/day)

The diet for an individual with diabetes can only be a dietary prescription based on nutrition assessment and treatment goals. The diabetic renal diet can be a good guideline to control and manage diabetes mellitus, which may then go into renal diseases.

RENAL DIET – THE MEALS

The following diet is divided by:

Breakfast

Lunch

Dinner

Desserts

Extra and minimal meals for different moments of the day.

You will have a list of ingredients, a paragraph dedicated to "how to prepare" the recipe and a list of nutrients per portion.

All recipes, divided by the different moments of the day, are listed in alphabetic order.

BREAKFAST

AVOCADO TOAST WITH EGGS

Ingredients
2 slices of whole-grain bread

1 tablespoon of parsley

½ Hass avocado

1 tablespoon of lime juice

1/8 teaspoon salt

2 eggs

2 tablespoons of crumbled feta cheese

1/8 teaspoon of ground black pepper

How to prepare the recipe
Toast the bread slices and cut the parsley into thin cubes or slices, setting it apart.

Mash half of avocado with a fork after you have removed the skin and add lime juice and a bit of salt. Spread this mixture on the toast slices.

Prepare a dish to be put in the oven at medium heat by spreading it with non-stick cooking spray. Break the eggs in the dish and cook them until you are satisfied with their consistency. Put the eggs onto the top of the avocado on the toast and put some feta cheese on the eggs, add the chopped parsley and the ground black pepper.

Nutrients per portion

225 calories

12 g protein

15 g carbohydrates

13 g fat

195 mg cholesterol

404 mg sodium

311 mg potassium

209 mg phosphorus

107 mg calcium

4.3 fiber

ASPARAGUS AND CHEESE
CREPES WITH PARSLEY

Ingredients

12 asparagus

4 ounces of soft cheese

1/2 teaspoon of black pepper

1/3 cup of flour

½ glass of water

¼ bowl of cream

1 egg

2 egg whites

4 tablespoons of butter

1 piece of parsley

1 teaspoon of lemon juice

How to prepare the recipe

Cook the asparagus for 6 to 8 minutes

Mix the softened cream cheese with the parsley, spices and lemon juice to prepare a sauce.

Put then together flour with water, egg, egg whites, and 2 tablespoons of butter already melted: mix everything to prepare a batter.

Prepare 8 to 10-inch crepe by melting the butter taken from 1/2 tablespoon, adding 1/3 of cup crepe batter and turn the pan to spread the batter. Cook it on both sides, cool it and repeat in order to prepare 4 crepes. Insert the cheese in the crepes that you are willing to roll afterward, putting inside also the asparagus.

Put them in the fridge for 1 hour, and after cut the crepes rolls into 3-4 pieces before putting them on the table.

Nutrients per portion

305 calories

10 g protein

16 g carbohydrates

24 g fat

114 mg cholesterol

245 mg sodium

355 mg potassium

140 mg phosphorus

95 mg calcium

2.8 fiber

BAKED FRENCH TOAST IN BATTER

Ingredients

4 slices Italian bread

4 cups of non-enriched rice milk

2 cups liquid low cholesterol egg substitute

½ cup sugar

4 spoons unsalted margarine (tablespoons)

1 teaspoon almond extract

1 teaspoon cinnamon

Non-calories sweetener

How to prepare the recipe

Spread margarine or non-stick cooking spray in the pan on the bottom and sides of it.

Put sliced bread on the bottom of the pan

Beat non-enriched rice milk, egg substitute, melted margarine, sugar, almond extract, and cinnamon all together in a cup and pour over bread slices.

Cover everything with plastic wrap and put it in the fridge for one night.

 Preheat oven at 350°F (around 170 é Celsius)

Bake for 50 minutes until the knife can cut easily and serve warm.

Sprinkle with non-calories sweetener if you wish.

Nutrients per portion

450 calories

16 g protein

65 g carbohydrates

14 g fat

0 mg cholesterol

390 mg sodium

220 mg potassium

110 mg phosphorus

86 mg calcium

0.8 fiber

BENEDICTS' EGGS MUFFINS

Ingredients

4 ounces of bacon in slices

3 glasses of water

2 muffins

1 tablespoon vinegar

1 tablespoon of lemon juice

4 eggs

1/2 cup of unsalted butter

3 egg yolks

pepper

paprika

How to prepare the recipe

Place the bacon in 2 cups of boiling water for 5 minutes in order to demineralize it. Put it on a towel and dry it to absorb the moisture. Cut the muffins and toast them. Cut the bacon and place it on top of each muffin slice. Put vinegar with water in a big bowl and boil it, reducing the heat slowly.

Break the eggs and put them into the water to poach them. Cover and wait for 3 to 5 minutes for the eggs to be ready. Remove the eggs and put them on the bacon and muffin, cover it and keep it warm.

At a light heat beat the yolks and melt some butter, adding this to the eggs with paprika and pepper. Add some lemon juice and pour all on top of the muffins.

Nutrients per portion

415 calories

15 g protein

15 g carbohydrates

35 g fat

440 mg cholesterol

345 mg sodium

170 mg potassium

214 mg phosphorus

105 mg calcium

1.0 fiber

BLUEBERRY SMOOTHIE

Ingredients

1 cup of frozen blueberries

2 tablespoons of whey protein powder

¼ of Greek yogurt, non-fat yogurt

1/3 cup unsweetened vanilla with almond milk

2 strawberries

5 raspberries

1 tablespoon of fiber cereals

2 teaspoons of shredded coconut

How to prepare the recipe

Put the blueberries in a blender for 1 minute, add yogurt, protein powder and milk, blend all together until it is soft and scoop the mixture into a bowl.

Top everything with sliced strawberries, raspberries, fiber cereals and shredded coconut. Add honey if you like it or a sweetener.

Nutrients per portion

225 calories

15 g protein

28 g carbohydrates

5 g fat

3 mg cholesterol

118 mg sodium

370 mg potassium

175 mg phosphorus

240 mg calcium

7.8 fiber

CEREALS AND RICE CAKES MIX

Ingredients

1cup of corn cereals

1 cup rice cereals

1/2 cup Cocoa cereals

1/2 cup of mini rice cakes (plain or apple cinnamon)

How to prepare the recipe

In a medium container mix all ingredients together and prepare separate portions.

Serve dry or with milk substitute.

Ask your doctor for a list of approved cereals.

Nutrients per portion

145 calories

2 g protein

32 g carbohydrates

1 g fat

0 mg cholesterol

235 mg sodium

70 mg potassium

50 mg phosphorus

96 mg calcium

1.0 fiber

EASY CREPE

Ingredients

3 eggs

1-1/3 whole milk

¾ all-purpose white flour

3 tablespoon butter

How to prepare the recipe

Mix both eggs and milk in a blender.

Add flour slowly and blend for 1 minute

Pour crepe batter in a bowl and add melted butter.

Heat a 8 inches crepe pan and coat pan with butter or non-stick cooking spray all at medium heat.

Pour batter into the pan and make sure it lies evenly moving the pan if necessary. The crepe will bubble.

Remove from pan when the crepe is golden, and its edges are a bit brown.

Nutrients per portion

60 calories

3 g protein

6 g carbohydrates

3 g fat

46 mg cholesterol

29 mg sodium

50 mg potassium

45 mg phosphorus

31 mg calcium

0.1 fiber

EGG CUPS

Ingredients

6 slices low sodium bacon

1/3 cup onion

1/3 cup mushrooms

1/3 cup bell pepper

12 large eggs

¼ teaspoon black pepper

How to prepare the recipe

Preheat the oven at 350°F. Line muffin tin with paper muffin wrappers. Bake bacon until it crisps. In a big bowl, crumble cooked bacon and mix it with dices of vegetables. Put the mixture into different cups, filling them by 2/3, leaving room to add the mixture itself. In another recipient beat together both eggs and black pepper.

Pour egg mixture into each muffin cup. Leave ¼ inch at the top.

Bake 25 minutes until muffin has risen and are firm. Remove them from the pan and serve.

Nutrients per portion

80 calories

7 g protein

1 g carbohydrates

5 g fat

210 mg cholesterol

80 mg sodium

90 mg potassium

100 mg phosphorus

28 mg calcium

0.1 fiber

FRENCH TOAST WITH CINNAMON APPLE

Ingredients

1 pound loaf cinnamon

8 ounces crème cheese

1 or 2 apples

6 tablespoon unsalted butter

1 teaspoon ground cinnamon

8 eggs

1 e ¼ cup half and half creamer

1 e ¼ cup almond milk, unsweetened

¼ cup pancake syrup

How to prepare the recipe

Divide both bread and cream cheese into dices. Remove peel and cut the apples into small cubes. Melt the butter.

Coat a 9" x 13" baking dish with cooking spray. Place half of the sliced bread into the dish and sprinkle the cream cheese dices over the bread, topping it with apple cubes. Spread the cinnamon on top with the rest of the bread.

In a pie dish beat the eggs with the half and half creamer, the milk, melted butter, and pancake syrup. Pour the mixture over the bread.

Cover your cooking dish with plastic wrap and press so that all the pieces are soaked. Refrigerate for 2 hours at least.

Preheat the oven at 325° F. Bake for 50 minutes and let it stand afterward for at least 10 minutes before serving. You can cut it into squares for up to 12 portions.

Put the pancake syrup on and add jam or cinnamon/raspberry applesauce if you like it.

Nutrients per portion

320 calories

9 g protein

27 carbohydrates

20 g fat

170 mg cholesterol

280 mg sodium

224 mg potassium

150 mg phosphorus

116 mg calcium

1.8 fiber

GRAPEFRUIT IN BROILED HONEY

Ingredients

1 grapefruit

2 teaspoons of honey

¼ teaspoon cinnamon

How to prepare the recipe

Preheat the broiler at 300°F (that is 150°Celsius)

Cut your grapefruit in half and cut it in the form of a semicircle

Drizzle the top of each grapefruit with honey and 1/8 teaspoon of cinnamon

Broil it for 6 minutes until it starts to brown and serve it hot.

Nutrients per portion

6 calories

1 g protein

17 carbohydrates

0 g fat

0 mg cholesterol

1 mg sodium

175 mg potassium

1 mg phosphorus

20 mg calcium

1.2 fiber

HASH BROWN OMELET

Ingredients

2 tablespoons of diced onion

1 teaspoon of canola oil

2 tablespoons of shredded hash brown

2 tablespoons of diced fresh green bell pepper

1 egg

2 tablespoons soy milk

2 egg whites

2 pieces of parsley

How to prepare the recipe

Heat oil at medium heat and add the diced onion pieces and green pepper, cooking it for 2 minutes.

Add hash brown and cook it or heat it (if not frozen) for 5 minutes.

Meanwhile, beat the eggs with soy milk and add nondairy creamer.

Pour the eggs in a pan and cook them to prepare an omelet until it is ready and firm. Place the hash brown on the omelet in the middle and roll it on a plate.

Add parsley and spices.

Nutrients per portion

225 calories

15 g protein

12 g carbohydrates

13 g fat

165 mg cholesterol

180 mg sodium

305 mg potassium

128 mg phosphorus

38 mg calcium

0.9 fiber

OMELET WITH APPLE AND ONION

Ingredients

3 eggs

1 water tablespoon

1 butter tablespoon

1 apple

¼ cup of low-fat milk

1/8 tablespoon of black pepper

2 small spoons of cheddar cheese

¾ cup sweet onion

How to prepare the recipe

Peel the apple and slice thinly both apple and onion

Pre heat the over at 400° F (that is around 200°C)

Prepare a small bowl and put in it both water, eggs
with milk, pepper, and leave it there. Melt the butter
over medium heat. Add apple and onion and wait
until the onion becomes translucent for about 5 - 6
minutes. Spread the mix of onion and apple in the
bowl and put the egg mixture over medium heat until
the edges set. Then add cheddar over the top and put
the skillet in the oven for about 10 minutes.

Divide the omelet into two parts and put it on a plate,
serving it immediately.

Nutrients per portion

284 calories

13 g protein

20 carbohydrates

15 g fat

300 mg cholesterol

165 mg sodium

340 mg potassium

23 mg phosphorus

145 mg calcium

3.5 fiber

ROLL UP BURRITO

Ingredients

4 eggs

3 tablespoons of green chiles

½ teaspoon of pepper sauce

¼ teaspoon ground cumin

2 flour tortillas in burrito size

Non-stick cooking spray

How to prepare the recipe

Put the non-stick cooking spray in a pan and heat a medium heat.

Beat eggs with green chiles, cumin and hot pepper sauce. Put the eggs into the pan and cook them for 2 minutes.

Heat tortillas in a skillet at medium heat. Place half the eggs mix on each tortilla and roll up.

Nutrients per portion

366 calories

18 g protein

30 g carbohydrates

18 g fat

370 mg cholesterol

590 mg sodium

245 mg potassium

300 mg phosphorus

115 mg calcium

2.5 fiber

VANILLA WAFFLES

Ingredients

2 eggs

2 glasses of cake flour

¾ glass of low-fat milk

¾ teaspoons of baking soda

¾ cup of sour cream

6 tablespoons of powdered sugar

4 tablespoons of unsalted butter

2 teaspoons of vanilla extract

2 tablespoons of granulated sugar

How to prepare the recipe

Heat the waffle iron

Put together the cake flour and baking soda.

Separate egg whites and yolks. Mix together egg yolks, sour cream, milk and vanilla.

Melt the butter and put it into the sour cream mix.

In another cup beat the egg whites with a hand mixer on medium speed until the peak is soft and add granulated sugar to the egg whites, still beating until stiff peaks form for 3 or 4 minutes.

Beat the sour cream mixture into the flour mix until they combine and then add the egg whites to smooth everything .

Add the batter to the waffle iron, close and cook for about 3-4 minutes. Serve waffles with powder sugar on it or top it with fresh berries, jam, syrup or whipped cream.

Nutrients per portion

367 calories

8 g protein

50 carbohydrates

15 g fat

98 mg cholesterol

200 mg sodium

150 mg potassium

120 mg phosphorus

80 mg calcium

1 g fiber

YOGURT FANTASY

Ingredients

Greek yogurt

1 spoon of vanilla whey protein powder

½ cup blueberries

How to prepare the recipe

Add protein powder to the yogurt slowly and mix after each addition. Do not mix all at once or it may be clumpy. Wash the blueberries and dry them. Place on top of the yogurt mixture.

Nutrients per portion

185 calories

25 g protein

19 carbohydrates

2 g fat

45 mg cholesterol

122 mg sodium

334 mg potassium

215 mg phosphorus

183 mg calcium

1.8 fiber

LUNCH

FRESH CUCUMBER SOUP

Ingredients

2 cucumbers

1/3 cup white onion

1 green onion

1/4 cup fresh mint

2 tablespoons fresh lemon juice

2 tablespoons fresh dill

2/3 cup water

1/3 cup sour cream

1/2 cup half and half cream

1/2 teaspoon pepper

1/4 teaspoon salt

How to prepare the recipe

Remove both peel and seeds from cucumbers.

Cut mint and the onions. Cut up dill.

Put all ingredients in a mixer and whisk until smooth

Cover and place in the refrigerator for at least 2 hour

Use fresh dill sprigs to garnish the soup

Nutrients per portion

78 calories

2 g protein

5 g carbohydrates

5 g fat

11 mg cholesterol

127 mg sodium

257 mg potassium

65 mg phosphorus

BERRY SALAD WITH
ITALIAN RICOTTA CHEESE

Ingredients

1 cup of fresh blackberries

1 cup of fresh blueberries

2 cups of fresh strawberry

1/3 cup lemon juice

2 cups of fresh Italian ricotta cheese

1/8 teaspoon of cinnamon

How to prepare the recipe

Wash well both blackberries and blueberries and strawberries. Slice them and put them all together. Add some lemon juice from the cup.

Put the ricotta cheese on a round plate or a bowl and then cover it with berries. Spread the cinnamon on it.

Nutrients per portion

140 calories

15 g protein

15 g carbohydrates

2 g fat

15 mg cholesterol

380 mg sodium

350 mg potassium

180 mg phosphorus

125 mg calcium

4.3 fiber

CELERY TUNA SALAD

Ingredients

1 piece of celery

15 ounces packed and unsalted tuna

½ apple

½ small onion

2 tablespoons mayonnaise

a bit of black pepper

a little bit of salt

How to prepare the recipe

Prepare the tuna and cut the apple, celery and onion.

Mix all together adding mayonnaise, black pepper and if you wish some salt.

Serve on lettuce and with unsalted crackers

Nutrients per portion

20 calories

27 g protein

3 g carbohydrates

9 g fat

35 mg cholesterol

185 mg sodium

318 mg potassium

183 mg phosphorus

20 mg calcium

0.8 fiber

MEAT CASSEROLE

Ingredients

10 ounces of reduced-fat pork sausage

8 ounces of cream cheese

1 glass of low-fat milk

4 slices of white bread

5 eggs

½ teaspoon dry mustard

½ dry onion flakes

How to prepare the recipe

Preheat oven at 325°F (160°C). Cut the sausage and cook in a cooking dish. Set aside and mix all other ingredients. Add cooked sausage to mixture and place bread pieces in a square casserole, pour sausage mix over the bread and cook for 50 minutes. Cut into 10 portions and serve

Nutrients per portion

222 calories

10 g protein

9 g carbohydrates

15 g fat

145 mg cholesterol

355 mg sodium

200 mg potassium

156 mg phosphorus

96 mg calcium

0.4 fiber

RED AND GREEN GRAPES
CHICKEN SALAD WITH CURRY

Ingredients

1 apple

1/4 bowl seedless red grapes

1/4 bowl seedless green grapes

4 cooked skinless and boneless chicken breasts

1 piece of celery

1/2 bowl of onion

1/2 bowl of canned water chestnuts

1/2 teaspoon curry powder

3/4 cup mayonnaise

1/8 teaspoon black pepper

How to prepare the recipe

Cut the chicken into small dices and chop celery, onion and apple. Drain and cut chestnuts. Put together the chicken pieces, celery, onion, apple, grapes, water chestnuts, pepper, curry powder and mayonnaise. Serve it in a big salad bowl.

Nutrients per portion

235 calories

13 g protein

6 g carbohydrates

18 g fat

44 mg cholesterol

160 mg sodium

200 mg potassium

115 mg phosphorus

15 mg calcium

1.1 fiber

GRILLED CHICKEN PIZZA

Ingredients

2 pita bread

3 tablespoons low sodium bbq sauce

¼ bowl red onion

4 ounces cooked chicken

2 tablespoons crumbled feta cheese

1/8 teaspoon garlic powder

How to prepare the recipe

Pre heat oven at 350°F (that is 175° C). Place 2 pitas on the pan after you have put non-stick cooking spray on it. Spread bbq sauce (2 tablespoons) on the pita. Cut the onion and put it on pita. Cube chicken and put it on the pitas. Put also both feta and the garlic powder over the pita. Bake for 12 minutes.

Nutrients per portion

320 calories

22 g protein

35 g carbohydrates

9 g fat

50 mg cholesterol

520 mg sodium

250 mg potassium

220 mg phosphorus

160 mg calcium

2.0 fiber

GROUND BEEF LOAN IN A CUP

Ingredients

¼ pound ground beef

2 tablespoons of low-fat milk

2 teaspoons of ketchup

2 tablespoons of quick-cooking oats

1 teaspoon onion powder

How to prepare the recipe

Spray a large cup with non-stick cooking spray.

 In another cup put together the milk (or its substitute), ketchup, onion, oats.ù

Crumble meat over the mixture and mix everything, pressing the ground beef.

Cover and put it in the microwave for 3 minutes (high) and serve it very warm.

Nutrients per portion

250 calories

25 g protein

13 g carbohydrates

10 g fat

75 mg cholesterol

160 mg sodium

395 mg potassium

245 mg phosphorus

65 mg calcium

1.4 fiber

MEXICAN BEEF FLOUR WRAP

Ingredients

5 ounces of cooked roast beef

8 cucumber slices

2 flour Tortillas 6" size

2 tablespoons of whipped cream cheese

2 leaves of light green lettuce

¼ of a bowl of cut red onion

¼ of stripped cut sweet bell pepper

1 teaspoon of herb seasoning blend

How to prepare the recipe

Spread the cheese over the flour wraps. Try to use the ingredients to make two wraps.

Layer the tortillas with roast beef, onions, lettuce, pepper strips and cucumber.

Sprinkle with the herb seasoning. Roll up the wraps and cut them into 4 pieces each. Serve fresh.

Nutrients per portion

255 calories

24 g protein

18 g carbohydrates

10 g fat

70 mg cholesterol

275 mg sodium

445 mg potassium

250 mg phosphorus

58 mg calcium

1.6 fiber

MIXED CHORIZO IN EGG FLOUR WRAPS

Ingredients

1 pack of chorizo

1 egg

1 flour tortilla or 6" size

How to prepare the recipe

Cook the chorizo in a pan on stove, cutting the meat into small pieces.

Eliminate excessive water or fat and add 1 egg combining all while they are being cooked.

Serve everything on a flour tortilla or wrapping the tortillas.

Nutrients per portion

223 calories

15 g protein

15 g carbohydrates

11 g fat

210 mg cholesterol

315 mg sodium

285 mg potassium

230 mg phosphorus

78 mg calcium

1.5 fiber

SANDWICH WITH CHICKEN SALAD

Ingredients

2 bowls of cooked chicken

½ cup of low-fat mayonnaise

½ cup of green bell pepper

1 cup of pieces of pineapple

1/3 cup of carrots

4 slices of flatbread

½ teaspoon of black pepper

How to prepare the recipe

Prepare aside the diced chicken and drain pineapple, adding green bell pepper , black pepper and carrots. Combine all in a bowl and refrigerate until chilled. Later on, serve the chicken salad on the flatbread.

Nutrients per portion

345 calories

22 g protein

24 g carbohydrates

15 g fat

60 mg cholesterol

395 mg sodium

330 mg potassium

165 mg phosphorus

15 mg calcium

1.5 fiber

SPICE BREAD WITH TUNA SALAD

Ingredients

1 tablespoon of onion

1 piece of celery

1 fresh tomato

Some lettuce leaves

1 tablespoon low calories mayonnaise

1 medium bagel or spiced bread

½ pack low sodium of water-packed canned tuna

How to prepare the recipe

Chop onion, tomato and celery. Open tuna and cut it into small pieces. Put everything in the bagel on the lettuce leaves adding some mayonnaise and close the spiced bread.

Nutrients per portion

290 calories

25 g protein

30 g carbohydrates

7 g fat

20 mg cholesterol

475 mg sodium

320 mg potassium

175 mg phosphorus

15 mg calcium

2.5 g fiber

SMOOTHIE WITH LEMON

Ingredients

4 teaspoons of sugar substitute

2 teaspoons of lemon juice

3 tablespoons whipped topping

8 ounces pasteurized liquid egg white

How to prepare the recipe

Put together all ingredients. Mix until the topping melts together well.

Nutrients per portion

225 calories

28 g protein

22 g carbohydrates

3 g fat

0 mg cholesterol

425 mg sodium

430 mg potassium

35 mg phosphorus

19 mg calcium

0 g fiber

STUFFED OMELET

Ingredients

2 tablespoons of red bell chopped pepper

2 tablespoons of orange bell chopped pepper

2 tablespoons of chopped green onion

2 tablespoons of fresh sliced mushrooms

1 teaspoon of chopped garlic

1 tablespoon butter

1 tablespoon canola oil

2 eggs

2 egg whites

4 tablespoon 1% low-fat milk

1/8 teaspoon ground cumin

1/8 teaspoon pepper

How to prepare the recipe

Pass the vegetables with garlic in butter or in oil mixture until they are tenderly crispy. Mix up eggs, egg whites and milk until they are light and tender as well. Mix it in cumin and pepper and pour egg mixture over the vegetables.

Reduce heat and cover for 1 to 2 minutes. Uncover and after egg is completely cooked, fold omelet over in the pan. Divide the omelet into 2 portions and serve. You can also garnish with green onion or a mushroom slice.

Nutrients per portion

220 calories

12 g protein

4 g carbohydrates

1 g fat

203 mg cholesterol

185 mg sodium

245 mg potassium

145 mg phosphorus

81 mg calcium

1.0 fiber

TINY RICE PIES

Ingredients

Vegetable oil (2 tablespoons)

1 teaspoon of mustard seeds

Half cup of semolina

2 green finely cut chilies

1/8 teaspoon salt

¼ cup of yogurt

¼ glass of water

¼ grated corn

¼ Indian cheese

Some bits of finely cut cilandro

1 tablespoon of clarified butter

How to prepare the recipe

Heat the oil and the seeds in a pan and add semolina, chilies and a bit of salt. Cook it until the semolina becomes a bit brown. Let it cool down. Put together yogurt with some water and mix it until it is smooth, then add corn, Indian cheese, cilantro, yogurt and add everything to semolina, leaving it aside for 10-15 minutes.

Put the clarified butter in a pan, steaming then the semolina mix for 10 minutes.

Put some cilantro on the semolina circles and serve
them still a bit warm.

Nutrients per portion

175 calories

5 g protein

14 g carbohydrates

10 g fat

4 mg cholesterol

214 mg sodium

140 mg potassium

89 mg phosphorus

65 mg calcium

0.8 fiber

TOAST TOPPED WITH CREAMY EGGS

Ingredients

4 slices white bread

6 eggs

4 ounces cream cheese

3 tablespoons of unsalted butter

1/3 cup flour

1-1/2 cups unsweetened, plain almond milk

1/2 tablespoon of yellow mustard

1/8 teaspoon pepper

How to prepare the recipe

Hard boil the eggs for 12 minutes. Remove them from heat, drain and cover with cool water. Peel and chop boiled eggs. Put together the butter and flour in a sauce pan at medium low heat. Mix constantly until well combined.

Add almond milk, cream cheese, mustard and pepper to butter and flour mixture. Let it thicken and add the eggs to the sauce, keeping at a warm heat. Toast the bread and put the egg mixture over the toast before serving.

Nutrients per portion

430 calories

15 g protein

25 g carbohydrates

28 g fat

330 mg cholesterol

400 mg sodium

250 mg potassium

210 mg phosphorus

220 mg calcium

1.6 fiber

DINNER

CHICKEN WITH VEGETABLES AND WORCESTERSHIRE SAUCE

Ingredients
1 cup of frozen sliced carrots

1 cup of frozen green beans

½ cup of diced onion

1 pound chicken breasts (boneless and skinless)

½ cup low sodium chicken consommé

Worcestershire sauce (2 teaspoons)

1 small spoon of herb seasoning

How to prepare the recipe
Put together carrots, green beans and onion in a pan and cook them slowly. Put the chicken breasts on vegetables and pour the consommé over the chicken. Top with Worcestershire sauce and herb seasoning.

Cook at a high heat for 3 hours or low heat for 6 hours.

Serve the chicken accompanied by the consommé in a cup and the vegetable mix.

Nutrients per portion

180 calories

25 g protein

10 g carbohydrates

3 g fat

70 mg cholesterol

185 mg sodium

430 mg potassium

225 mg phosphorus

55 mg calcium

3.2 fiber

GROUND BEEF SOUP

Ingredients

Lean ground beef cut in small balls (1 pound)

½ glass of onion

1 small spoon seasoning and browning sauce

2 small spoons of lemon pepper seasoning blend

Some reduced-sodium beef consommé

2 glasses of water

Half dish white rice

Half pack of frozen mixed vegetables (corn, carrots, peas, beans and green beans)

Half spoon of sour cream

How to prepare the recipe

Brown ground beef with cut onion in a pan and eliminate fat. Add seasoning sauce, water, consommé, rice and vegetables. On high heat boil the ingredients and after lowering the heat, cook for 30 minutes.

Put the meatballs in the consommé and cook at a low heat still for half an hour until ready to serve.

Nutrients per portion

220 calories

20 g protein

18 g carbohydrates

8 g fat

50 mg cholesterol

170 mg sodium

445 mg potassium

210 mg phosphorus

42 mg calcium

4.2 fiber

GROUND TURKEY BURGER

Ingredients

1 pound ground lean turkey

6 hamburger buns

½ dish red onion

½ dish of green bell pepper

1 half spoon of chicken grilled blend seasoning

2 small spoons of brown sugar

1 tablespoon Worcestershire sauce

1 cup of low sodium tomato sauce

How to prepare the recipe

Cook the turkey at medium heat. Cut little pieces of onion and green bell pepper. Mix the sauce, the grilled blend seasoning and tomato sauce. Add seasoning to the turkey mixture and cook for 10 minutes. Prepare 5 portions and put in burger buns.

Nutrients per portion

28 calories

24 g protein

28 g carbohydrates

9 g fat

55 mg cholesterol

285 mg sodium

510 mg potassium

235 mg phosphorus

85 mg calcium

1.8 fiber

ONE PORTION FRITTATAS

Ingredients

4 eggs

2 tablespoons red bell pepper

2 tablespoons green bell pepper

2 tablespoons onion

2 ounces cooked lean ham

1 tablespoon low-fat milk

1 pound frozen hash brown potatoes

½ bowl low-fat cheddar cheese

Black pepper

How to prepare the recipe

Put the potatoes in water in a bowl for 4 hours. Eliminate excessive water.

Pre heat oven at 375°F (or 200°C). Coat 8 muffin tins holes with cooking spray. Put hash brown potatoes in the tins and press them in the bottom then spray also the potatoes with cooking spray. Cook for 12-15 minutes at 350°F (175° C). Cut the ham, pepper and onion finely and beat both milk and eggs together in a bowl. Season with pepper and add ham, pepper, onion and cheese to the mixture.

Put the hash brown potatoes in the muffin holes pressing them and out ¼ bowl egg mixture in the center of each muffin hole. Put again the pan in the oven and let the potatoes become crispy in about 15 to 20 minutes.

Once ready, let the muffins sit on a dish for 5 minutes before serving.

Nutrients per portion

110 calories

8 g protein

10 g carbohydrates

4 g fat

100 mg cholesterol

115 mg sodium

160 mg potassium

130 mg phosphorus

52 mg calcium

1.0 fiber

PAN FRIED BEEF AND BROCCOLI

Ingredients

2 garlic small slices

1 tomato

8 ounces uncooked lean sirloin beef

12 ounces of frozen broccoli stir fry vegetable blend

2 little spoons of peanut oil

¼ cup low sodium chicken consommé

1 small spoon of cornstarch

2 little spoons of reduced-sodium soy sauce

2 bowls of cooked rice

How to prepare the recipe

Cut the garlic cloves and tomato. Cut the beef into strips and place the broccoli in the microwave for 3-4 minutes. In a wok pan heat oil and the garlic to make them fragrant. Add vegetable blend cooking it for about 4 minutes or more and remove from pan.

Add the beef in the same pot and cook it for around 7-8 minutes, then prepare the sauce putting together the consommé, the soy sauce and cornstarch.

Add vegetables, sauce, tomato and heat them with the beef until the sauce is ready. Serve the dish with brown rice.

Nutrients per portion

370 calories

18 g protein

35 g carbohydrates

17 g fat

40 mg cholesterol

350 mg sodium

550 mg potassium

250 mg phosphorus

60 mg calcium

5.1 fiber

PORK CHOPS AND APPLES

Ingredients

Unsalted margarine (2 tablespoons)

6 ounces of low sodium stuffing mix for chicken

20 ounces apple pie filling

6 boneless pork loin chops

Olive oil

How to prepare the recipe

Put a baking pan in the oven at 350°F (or 200°C) and grease it with olive oil.

Put together the stuffing and mix it in water and margarine. Spread the apple pie pieces on the bottom of the pan and place pork chops on it. Put the stuffing on top of pork chops.

Cover with parchment paper and bake for 30 minutes. Remove the paper and still leave it in the oven for 10 minutes.

Nutrients per portion

490 calories

25 g protein

45 g carbohydrates

20 g fat

55 mg cholesterol

365 mg sodium

405 mg potassium

220 mg phosphorus

25 mg calcium

1.0 fiber

RIGATONI SPRING PASTA

Ingredients

12 ounces of rigatoni pasta (you can also use fusilli or farfalle pasta)

12 ounces vegetables (carrots, broccoli and zucchini or any other fresh vegetable)

2 portions of half and half creamer

Grated parmesan cheese

How to prepare the recipe

Boil the water and when the water gets to making bubbles put the pasta in it. For Rigatoni it will take around 11 minutes to cook. In the meantime put the cut and diced vegetables into a pan with some olive oil in it. Mix the vegetables until they are soft and ready, adding the two small portions of half and half creamer.

When the pasta boils, drain it in a strainer and put it in the pan where you have prepared the vegetables. Mix everything together and put the pasta on a dish, adding some parmesan cheese on top. (If you prefer you can add the parmesan cheese when you are mixing the ingredients in the pan at a medium heat). Then serve hot.

Nutrients per portion

253 calories

10 g protein

47 g carbohydrates

3 g fat

6 mg cholesterol

115 mg sodium

250 mg potassium

153 mg phosphorus

92 mg calcium

4.5 fiber

SALAD WITH STRAWBERRIES
AND GOAT CHEESE

Ingredients
Abundant baby lettuce
1 pint strawberries
Balsamic vinegar
Extra virgin olive oil
¼ teaspoon of black pepper
8 ounces soft goat cheese

How to prepare the recipe
Prepare the lettuce by washing and drying it, then cut the strawberries. Cut the soft goat cheese into 8 pieces. Put together the balsamic vinegar and the extra virgin olive oil in a large cup with a whisk.
Mix the strawberries pressing them and putting them in a bowl, add the dressing and mix, then divide the lettuce into four dishes and cut the other strawberries, arranging them on the salad. Put cheese slices on top and add pepper.

Nutrients per portion

300 calories

13 g protein

11 g carbohydrates

23 g fat

25 mg cholesterol

285 mg sodium

400 mg potassium

195 mg phosphorus

145 mg calcium

3.0 fiber

SALMON WITH SPICY HONEY

Ingredients

16 ounces of salmon fillet

3 tablespoons of honey

¾ little spoons of lemon peel

3 bowls of arugula salad

½ spoon of black pepper

½ spoon of garlic powder

2 small spoons of olive oil

1 teaspoon of hot water

How to prepare the recipe

Prepare a small bowl with some hot water and put in honey, grated lemon peel, ground pepper, garlic powder. Spread the mixture over salmon fillets.

Warm some olive oil at a medium heat and add spiced salmon fillet and cook for 4 minutes. Turn the fillets on one side then on the other side.

Continue to cook for other 4 minutes at a reduced heat and try to check when the salmon fillets flake easily . Put some arugula on each plate and add the salmon fillets on top, adding some aromatic herbs or some dill.

Nutrients per portion

320 calories

23 g protein

15 g carbohydrates

19 g fat

60 mg cholesterol

65 mg sodium

450 mg potassium

250 mg phosphorus

42 mg calcium

0.4 fiber

SPECIAL CHILI

Ingredients

1 pound ground lean beef

2 pounds turkey

1 onion

½ green bell pepper

2 garlic cloves

1 cumin seed spoon

Some salt (one teaspoon)

1 teaspoon ground oregano

Black pepper (1/2 teaspoon)

Paprika (1/2 teaspoon)

1 tablespoon of white flour

3 glasses of boiling water

¼ cup chili powder

6 ounces of tomato sauce (low sodium quality)

9 cups of white rice, cooked

How to prepare the recipe

Sauté beef and turkey in a pan until they are browned and add to the meat chopped onion, green pepper and garlic. Stir and add cumin, salt, oregano, pepper and paprika and stir again. Spread the flour over the mixture, mix with the boiling water and chili powder then stir and cook for one hour very slowly. Add tomato sauce and stir again. Cook for 30 minutes eliminating grease and serve hot with white rice.

Nutrients per portion

285 calories

25 g protein

35 g carbohydrates

13 g fat

75 mg cholesterol

300 mg sodium

550 mg potassium

275 mg phosphorus

50 mg calcium

2.3 fiber

STEW WITH BEEF AND BARLEY

Ingredients

1 bowl of uncooked barley in pearls

1 pound of lean beef stew meat

2 tablespoons of white flour

¼ teaspoon black pepper

½ teaspoon salt

2 little spoons of canola oil

2 small bits of onion

1 celery stalk

1 clove of garlic

2 carrots

2 bay leaves

1 bit of onion herb seasoning

How to prepare the recipe

Put the barley in a cup of water for 1 hour and dice both onion and celery. Add the garlic clove and slice the carrots. Cut beef into small cubes. Put the black pepper, flour and meat in a plastic bag shaking the ingredients. Heat on the stove and brown the stew meat. Remove meat from the pan. Brown and stir onion, celery and garlic for 2 minutes, add 2 quarts of water and bring to boil. Put back the meat to the pot and add bay leaves and salt, boiling slowly. Drain the barley and add to the pot, cover and cook for 1 hour. Blend every 15 minutes, then add carrots and herb seasoning. Blend for another hour and water every now and then in order not to let the ingredients stick.

Nutrients per portion

245 calories

20 g protein

20 g carbohydrates

8 g fat

50 mg cholesterol

220 mg sodium

365 mg potassium

175 mg phosphorus

30 mg calcium

6.2 fiber

STUFFED PEPPERS

Ingredients

4 bell peppers

1 tablespoon of dried parsley

2 cups of cooked white rice

2 small spoons of garlic powder

Black pepper (1 teaspoon)

¾ pound ground beef

½ bowl of chopped onion

3 ounces unsalted tomato sauce

How to prepare the recipe

Remove the seeds from black peppers

Preheat the oven at 375°F (or 200°C)

Roast the beef and add onion, rice, parsley, black pepper, garlic powder and tomato sauce to the beef. Boil slowly for 10 minutes. Feel the bell peppers with mixture and bake in the oven for one hour.

Nutrients per portion

260 calories

20 g protein

28 g carbohydrates

7 g fat

50 mg cholesterol

210 mg sodium

550 mg potassium

208 mg phosphorus

40 mg calcium

2.7 fiber

TURKEY SAUSAGES

Ingredients

¼ teaspoon salt

1/8 teaspoon garlic powder

1/8 teaspoon onion powder

1 teaspoon fennel seed

1 pound 7% fat ground turkey

How to prepare the recipe

Press the fennel seed and in a small cup put together turkey with fennel seed, garlic and onion powder and salt. Cover the bowl and refrigerate over night. Prepare the turkey with seasoning into different portions with a circle form and press them into patties ready to be cooked. Cook at a medium heat until browned. Cook it for 1 to 2 minutes per side and serve them hot.

Nutrients per portion

55 calories

7 g protein

0 g carbohydrates

3 g fat

24 mg cholesterol

70 mg sodium

105 mg potassium

75 mg phosphorus

9 mg calcium

0 fiber

VEGETARIAN PASTICCIO

Ingredients

7 eggs

7 slices of sourdough bread

1 ounce shredded sharp cheddar cheese

1 piece of onion

1 cup of raw mushrooms

1 cup red bell peppers

15 fresh spinach leaves

½ teaspoon black pepper

¼ glass vinegar§

3 portions of half and half cream

Worcestershire sauce (1 teaspoon)

Hot sauce (1 teaspoon)

Unsalted margarine (1 teaspoon)

How to prepare the recipe

Cut onion, pepper and mushrooms into small dices.

Chop bread into small dices and place on a baking sheet. Bake in the oven at 225°F (or 100°C) for 15 minutes, turning the cubes every 15 minutes and then still cook them for other 15 minutes.

Put onion, pepper and mushrooms mix in a skillet pre-greased with olive oil.

Grease a dish and put in it both bread dices and the vegetable mixture, then put the spinach leaves on top. Arrange for a second layer of the same mixture.

Put together the half and half cream with eggs, vinegar, Worcestershire sauce, hot sauce and black pepper. Pour this mix over the bread. Put the covered dish in the fridge for one hour. When out of the fridge, put the dish aside for at least 20 minutes.

Preheat oven at 325 °F (or 160°C). Bake for 50 minutes without the covering and when you take it out of the oven, sprinkle the cheddar cheese over the top. Cook for 10 minutes and cut into 10 slices and serve it hot.

Nutrients per portion

210 calories

10 g protein

15 g carbohydrates

10 g fat

165 mg cholesterol

215 mg sodium

345 mg potassium

205 mg phosphorus

150 mg calcium

2.0 fiber

ZUCCHINI AND CARROTS
ROSEMARY CHICKEN

Ingredients

2 zucchini

1 carrot

1 spoon of dried rosemary

4 chicken breasts

½ bell pepper

½ red onion

8 garlic cloves

Olive oil

¼ tablespoon ground pepper

How to prepare the recipe

Prepare the oven and preheat it at 375 °F (or 200°C). Slice both zucchini and carrots and add bell pepper, onion , garlic and put everything adding oil in a 13" x 9" pan. Spread the pepper over everything and roast for about 10 minutes.

Meanwhile, lift up the chicken skin and spread black pepper and rosemary on the flesh. Remove the vegetable pan from the oven and add the chicken, returning the pan to the oven for about 30 more minutes.

Nutrients per portion

215 calories

28 g protein

8 g carbohydrates

7 g fat

70 mg cholesterol

105 mg sodium

580 mg potassium

250 mg phosphorus

63 mg calcium

3.0 fiber

DESSERTS

APPLE OATMEAL CRUNCHY

Ingredients

5 Green apples

1 bowl of oatmeal

A small cup of brown sugar

1/2 cup of flour

1 teaspoon of cinnamon

½ bowl of butter

How to prepare the recipe

Prepare apples by cutting them in tiny slices and preheat the oven at 350°F.

In a cup mix oatmeal, flour, cinnamon and brown sugar. Put butter in the batter and place sliced apple in a baking pan (9" x 13").

Spread oatmeal mix over the apples and bake for 35 minutes.

Nutrients per portion

295 calories

3 g protein

40 g carbohydrates

12 g fat

30 mg cholesterol

95 mg sodium

190 mg potassium

73 mg phosphorus

35 mg calcium

2.3 fiber

APPLE CHUNKS PIE

Ingredients

2 apples

1 cup of unsalted butter

1 cup of brown sugar

1 cup of sour cream

1 teaspoon vanilla extract

1 teaspoon baking soda

½ spoon of salt

2 cups of flour

1 teaspoon of cinnamon

½ glass of milk

1 cup of powdered sugar

How to prepare the recipe

Preheat the oven (350°F or 200°C)

Cut the apples, put together half cup of butter with granulated sugar and brown sugar.

Add vanilla, sour cream, baking soda, salt and flour. Mix and add the apples.

Put everything in a pan (9"x 13") and then in the oven. In a small container mix 2 little spoons of butter, brown sugar and cinnamon. Spread on the top of the prepared batter and bake for 40 minutes. Let the pan cool and to make it icing add some butter, milk substitute and sugar on top, cutting the dessert in 18 or even 20 small chunks.

Nutrients per portion

245 calories

2 g protein

35 g carbohydrates

10 g fat

25 mg cholesterol

140 mg sodium

70 mg potassium

25 mg phosphorus

20 mg calcium

0.5 fiber

BERRY ICECREAM

Ingredients

6 ice cream cones

1 cup of whipped topping

1 cup of fresh blueberries

4 ounces cream cheese

¼ cup of blueberry jam

How to prepare the recipe

Put the cream cheese in a large cup and beat it with a mixer until it is fluffy. Mix with fruit and jam and whipped topping. Put the mixture on the small ice cream cones and refrigerate them in the freezer for 1 hour or more until they are ready to serve.

Nutrients per portion

175 calories

3 g protein

20 g carbohydrates

9 g fat

20 mg cholesterol

95 mg sodium

80 mg potassium

40 mg phosphorus

23 mg calcium

1 fiber

BUTTERMILK CAKE

Ingredients
1 buttermilk cup
1 deep dish of 9" pie crust
2 small spoons of lemon juice
2 eggs
¼ buttercup
1 small spoon of almond extract
1 teaspoon of vanilla extract
½ cup of sugar
4 small spoons of flour

How to prepare the recipe
In a large bowl mix together eggs, softened butter (pre-cooked and softened at 375°F), buttermilk, almond and vanilla extract, sugar and flour.

Put the mixture in a dish for pie crust and bake it for one hour. Leave it aside to cool and then serve it in slices.

Nutrients per portion

373 calories

4 g protein

45 g carbohydrates

18 g fat

85 mg cholesterol

145 mg sodium

90 mg potassium

65 mg phosphorus

45 mg calcium

0.2 fiber

CARAMEL PIE WITH APPLES

Ingredients

3 big apples

8 ounces of frozen dessert topping

2 caramel nut blast gold bars

How to prepare the recipe

Cut apples into small pieces and also cut caramel bars into small pieces.

Prepare whipped cream out of the fridge and mix it with caramel bar and apple pieces in a large bowl. Cool it for one hour before eating it.

Nutrients per portion

200 calories

5 g protein

25 g carbohydrates

10 g fat

0 mg cholesterol

45 mg sodium

115 mg potassium

45 mg phosphorus

40 mg calcium

1.5 fiber

CHERRY PIE

Ingredients

2 eggs

1 small cup of granulated sugar

Some sour cream

1 vanilla teaspoon

1/2 cup of unsalted butter

2 spoons of white flour

1 teaspoon of baking powder

1 teaspoon of baking soda

20 ounces of cherry pie filling or

10 cherries to be beaten and put in the cake

How to prepare the recipe

Use a mixer and make soft all together softened butter, sugar, eggs, vanilla and sour cream.

Preheat the oven at 350°F (or 200°C). in another bowl put together flour, baking powder, and baking soda.

Mix all together both dry and soft ingredients and pour the batter in a cooking dish for oven . You can disperse cherry pie filling or/and the cherries on the batter. Bake in the oven for 40 - 45 minutes.

Nutrients per portion

20 calories

3 g protein

30 g carbohydrates

8 g fat

42 mg cholesterol

110 mg sodium

70 mg potassium

70 mg phosphorus

40 mg calcium

0.5 fiber

CRANBERRY DESSERT

Ingredients

Cherry gelatine mix

Boiling water

12 ounces of cranberries

½ glass of sugar

12 ounces canned jelly cranberry sauce

12 ounces free whipped topping

How to prepare the recipe

Put the gelatine mix in the boiled hot water and set aside, letting it cool down. Put sugar in another boiling water. Then add the cranberries and boil for 5 minutes. When hot, remove the cranberries and add jellied cranberry sauce. Blend all together and break the jelly sauce into little chunks.

Add cool gelatine and whipped topping. Distribute topping throughout and removing it from the heat, cool it for one hour. Serve it cold.

Nutrients per portion

195 calories

1 g protein

35 g carbohydrates

5 g fat

0 mg cholesterol

35 mg sodium

30 mg potassium

10 mg phosphorus

4 mg calcium

1.5 fiber

CRUST PIE WITH CHERRY

Ingredients
1 box of sugar-free gelatine

1 pie crust

Light cream cheese

20 ounces no-sugar cherry pie filling

12 ounces frozen dessert whipped topping

How to prepare the recipe
Prepare the gelatine and put it in a pan refrigerating it to set.

Put out the cream cheese and let it soften, bake the pie crust and let it cool. Combine whipped topping and cream cheese until they are well together and soft. Cut gelatin into cubes and blend with the whipped topping mixture. Blend baked pie crust and spread the filling over the gelatine mixture.

Put in the fridge for 2 or 3 hours before serving.

Nutrients per portion

257 calories

5 g protein

25 g carbohydrates

13 g fat

10 mg cholesterol

213 mg sodium

150 mg potassium

50 mg phosphorus

30 mg calcium

1 fiber

LIME DESSERT

Ingredients

5 tablespoons extra virgin olive oil

1 and ¼ bowl of cracker crumbs

¼ glass granulated sugar

Lime juice

14 ounces canned sweetened condensed milk

1 small cup of heavy whipping cream

How to prepare the recipe

Pre heat oven at 350°F (or 175°C).

Blend olive oil, cracker crumbs and sugar, mix and save a pair of spoons to sprinkle in the end on top of the dessert.

Press the ingredients already mixed up in a 9" pie shell and bake for 5 minutes and cool it. Meanwhile add lime juice and mix with milk. Use a chilled bowl and whip the heavy cream to a stiff peak. Blend the cream with the condensed milk mixture.

Blend leftover crumb mixture on the dessert/pie. Chill and serve.

Nutrients per portion

425 calories

5 g protein

45 g carbohydrates

24 g fat

57 mg cholesterol

148 mg sodium

240 mg potassium

160 mg phosphorus

165 mg calcium

0.5 fiber

ORANGE AND ANISE COOKIES

Ingredients

White flour (2 cups)

2 teaspoons of baking powder

2 teaspoons of anise seed

1 teaspoon of grated orange peel

½ small cup of sugar

1 egg

2 tablespoons of canola oil

1 teaspoon orange extract

How to prepare the recipe

Preheat oven at 350°F (or 200 ° C). Line a large baking tray with baking paper.

Mix the dry ingredients in a large cup and blend, then place oil, egg and extract in a bowl and smooth, doing it either with a whisk or electric mixer for about 30 seconds.

Add the liquid and the dry mixture with a wooden spoon and prepare the dough by shaping it into a ball. Cut it in two parts and roll each half, then flatten it and place it on the cooking tray in the oven for about 20 minutes. Remove it and cut it with a bread knife to get around 18-20 cookies. Place them again in the oven for about 5 minutes. Remove them from the oven and cool on a rack.

Nutrients per portion

95 calories

2 g protein

15 g carbohydrates

2 g fat

10 mg cholesterol

45 mg sodium

25 mg potassium

75 mg phosphorus

42 mg calcium

0.5 fiber

PUDDING GLASS WITH BANANA
AND WHIPPED CREAM

Ingredients

2 portions of banana cream pudding mix

Rice milk (2,5 cups)

8 ounces dairy whipped cream

12 ounces vanilla wafers

How to prepare the recipe

Put vanilla wafers in a pan and in another bowl mix together banana cream pudding and rice milk. Boil the ingredients blending them slowly. Pour the mixture over the wafers and make 2 or 3 layers. Put the pan in the fridge for one hour and afterward spread the whipped topping over the dessert. Put it back in the fridge for 2 hours and serve it cool in transparent glasses.

Nutrients per portion

255 calories

3 g protein

45 g carbohydrates

7 g fat

3 mg cholesterol

275 mg sodium

50 mg potassium

40 mg phosphorus

8 mg calcium

0.3 fiber

PUMPKIN CHEESECAKE

Ingredients

1 egg white

1 wafer crumb 9" pie crust

½ small bowl of granulated sugar

Vanilla extract (1 teaspoon)

1 teaspoon of pumpkin pie flavoring

½ small bowl of liquid egg substitute

½ bowl of pumpkin cream

8 tablespoons of frozen topping for desserts

16 ounces cream cheese

How to prepare the recipe

Brush pie crust with egg white and cook for 5 minutes in a preheated oven from 375°F from 375°F now down to 350°F.

In a large cup put together sugar, vanilla and cream cheese, beating with a mixer until smooth. Beat the egg substitute and add pumpkin cream with pie flavoring: blend everything until softened.

Put the pumpkin mixture in a pie shell and bake for 50 minutes to set the center. Then let the pie cool down and then put it in the fridge. When you wish to, serve it in 8 slices putting some topping on it.

Nutrients per portion

364 calories

5 g protein

28 g carbohydrates

25 g fat

56 mg cholesterol

245 mg sodium

125 mg potassium

65 mg phosphorus

10 mg calcium

0.5 fiber

SMALL CHOCOLATE CAKES

Ingredients

1 box angel food cake mix

1 box lemon cake mix

Water

Non-stick cooking spray or butter

Dark Chocolate small squared chops and chocolate powder

How to prepare the recipe

Use a transparent kitchen cooking bag and put inside both lemon cake mix, angel food mix and chocolate chops. Mix everything together and add water to prepare a small cupcake. Put the mix in a mold to prepare a cupcake containing the ingredients and put in microwave for one-minute high temperature.

Slip the cupcake out of the mold and put it on a dish, let it cool and put some more chocolate crumbs on it.

Nutrients per portion

95 calories

1 g protein

21 g carbohydrates

1 g fat

0 mg cholesterol

162 mg sodium

15 mg potassium

80 mg phosphorus

20 mg calcium

0 fiber

STRAWBERRY WHIPPED CREAM CAKE

Ingredients

1 pint of whipping cream

2 tablespoons of gelatine

1/2 a glass of cold water

1 glass of boiling water

3 tablespoons of lemon juice

1 orange glass juice

1 spoon of sugar

¾ cup of sliced strawberries

1 large angel food cake or light sponge cake

How to prepare the recipe

Put the gelatine in cold water then add hot water and blend. Add orange and lemon juice, also add some sugar and go on blending. Refrigerate and leave it there until you see it is starting to gel.

Whip half portion of cream and add it to the mixture along with strawberries, put wax paper in the bowl and cut the cake in small pieces. In between the pieces, add the whipped cream and put everything in the fridge for one night.

When you take out the cake, add some whipped cream on top and decorate with some more fruit.

Nutrients per portion

355 calories

4 g protein

43 g carbohydrates

18 g fat

65 mg cholesterol

275 mg sodium

145 mg potassium

145 mg phosphorus

85 mg calcium

0.8 fiber

SWEET CRACKER PIE CRUST

Ingredients

1 bowl of graham cracker crumbs

¼ small cup of sugar

Unsalted butter

How to prepare the recipe

Mix sweet cracker crumbs, butter and sugar. Put in the over preheat at 375°F.

Bake for 7 minutes putting it in a greased pie. Let the pie cool before adding any kind of filling.

Nutrients per portion

205 calories

2 g protein

28 g carbohydrates

9 g fat

15 mg cholesterol

208 mg sodium

67 mg potassium

22 mg phosphorus

8 mg calcium

0.3 fiber